HAND THERAPY IN CHILDREN WITH CEREBRAL PALSY

A practical approach for parents, therapists and other healthcare professionals handling children with spastic cerebral palsy

PRIYA REDDAPPA

Hand Therapy in children with Cerebral Palsy

A practical approach for parents, therapists and other healthcare professionals handling children with spastic cerebral palsy

Author: Priya Reddappa

First Edition: 2019

Second Edition: 2025

ISBN: 978-93-342-8656-4

Published by: Priya Reddappa

Disclaimer: The information provided in this book is for educational purposes only and is based on the author's experience and research. This book is not intended to make any diagnosis or provide treatment for any medical condition. Please consult your primary care physician and therapist before beginning any exercise, or treatment provided in this book. The information in the book is to be followed or used after discussion with the therapist and under the therapist's care and supervision. The author and the publisher do not assume responsibility and are not liable to any party for any damages, loss, errors, injuries, or negative consequences resulting from reading or following the information provided in this book. The author and the publisher are not responsible for any health needs requiring medical supervision, increase in symptoms, or any health problem resulting from using the information in this book.

With the blessings of Shri Shirdi Sai Baba,

this work has been possible.

I dedicate this book to my family, whose love, support and

encouragement had been tremendous while

writing this book.

ABOUT THE AUTHOR

Priya Reddappa, MPT (Paediatric Neurology), APGDCR-PV, is a postgraduate Paediatric Physical Therapist, and a licensed Life Member of Indian Association of Physiotherapists (MIAP). She completed her Masters in Physical Therapy (Paediatric Neurology) from, The Tamilnadu Dr M.G.R Medical University and has experience as a Physical Therapist over 12 years in various clinical areas of Orthopaedics, Neurology, Cardiorespiratory, and Neuropaediatric conditions. As a clinically driven professional, she has worked in paediatric acute care (inpatient settings), outpatient settings, special school, and paediatric rehabilitation centers. She has handled paediatric patients at Apollo Children's Hospital, Chennai for over five years. She gained experience as a Research Clinical Evaluator for Apollo Hospitals Education and Research Foundation for a Clinical Trial on Duchenne Muscular Dystrophy for about four years. She has published two research papers in international journals regarding hand function in children with cerebral palsy, and adults with spinal cord injury. She has also published books on Physical therapy for hand function in children with cerebral palsy, Erb's palsy, and knee arthritis.

ACKNOWLEDGEMENT

I thank all the authors, whose books helped me, derive my knowledge during my graduation and apply them into my clinical practice for the last twelve years as a Paediatric Physical Therapist. I also thank the authors listed in the references at the end of this book, whose work has helped me to use the information to guide the readers of this book to further their knowledge into their practice and handling of children with cerebral palsy.

Priya Reddappa
Author

Table of Contents

CHAPTER 1: INTRODUCTION

Cerebral palsy is a set of neurological disorders that affects muscle movements, posture, (Koman & Smith, 2004) and coordination, appearing during the first two to three years of life. Cerebral palsy can result from multiple causes including severe hypoxia or ischemia at birth (MacLennan, Alastair H. et al. 2015). There is also an increased risk associated with preterm delivery, congenital malformations, multiple pregnancies, intrauterine infections, and placental abnormalities to cite a few.

Cerebral palsy has several subtypes including spasticity, ataxia, tremor, athetosis, and rigidity. A mixture of various movement disorders is common in cerebral palsy and they include hemiplegia, diplegia, triplegia, monoplegia, and quadriplegia. Spastic type of cerebral palsy is the most commonly occurring disorder. Children with cerebral palsy have poor development of hand function that involves individual finger movements (Pitroda, 2008). The general principles of management include reduction of spasticity, prevention and correction of deformities, strengthening antagonist's muscles and retraining functional patterns of movement (Terence et al, 2005).

The development of hand function is crucial for the infant and the young child to explore and interact with the surroundings. Impaired hand function interferes with the child's ability to carry on daily life activities and the child's socialization with peers. The development of hand skills in a child is associated with cognition (Exner, 2006). Play behaviour is compromised in children with hand dysfunction. Inhibiting spasticity will motivate the child to engage in play activities (Pfeifer et al, 2014). According to Illingworth (2007), "the development of manipulation is a better guide to the level of intelligence than is gross motor development." Only when we understand the normal development of hand function and the variations from the normal, we could identify and diagnose the abnormal (hand dysfunction) that has occurred in a child with cerebral palsy. Impaired manipulation skills also affect a child's academic performance and independence. The development of hand function is based on both the neurological and physical growth of a child. The child uses hands and arms to help and stabilize himself during various postures and to balance himself and avoid falls. The spastic type of cerebral palsy usually does not appear before eight months of life.

Every child with spastic type of cerebral palsy is unique in presentation. The classification as the spastic type of cerebral palsy may not happen until 8 months, though the child may be having developmental delay. Some children may appear as having a delay in development in their first few months which could either be just a delay or sometimes cerebral palsy or any other syndrome (there are many syndromes that present as developmental delay in children). The muscle tone of the child as spastic may appear late when the baby is around 8 months (in some cases may be evident earlier). The developmental milestones are not actually fixed but do vary from child to child. Some children with delay in development may later be diagnosed with cerebral palsy. Though the damage to the brain is non-progressive, the symptoms of the child may not be apparent in the first few months, because the different systems in the baby mature at different stages, the presentation of atypical changes in posture and movement, and of diagnosing the child with cerebral palsy may take time. The delay in the disappearance of the primitive reflexes and the delayed appearance of the postural reflex may be the initial indicator to diagnose a child regarding issues with posture and movement.

Neonates are born with reflex behaviour, which is automatic and helps them in arm and hand movements. These reflexes are integrated into voluntary movements when the baby reaches six months of age (Case-Smith, 2006).

This book deals with the improvement of hand function in children with spastic cerebral palsy who primarily have motor dysfunction. In the next chapter we shall know how the functions of the hand develop as the child grows.

CHAPTER 2: TYPICAL DEVELOPMENT OF HAND FUNCTION

TYPICAL DEVELOPMENT OF HAND FUNCTION DURING THE FIRST YEAR OF LIFE

During the second and third month of life, the baby develops neck righting reaction, with postural control. The eyes of the baby learn to scan the environment and develop spatiotemporal adaptation (Bole, 2007). The baby requires vestibular, proprioceptive, and visual-perceptual integration. When the baby is about three months old, it keeps its hands open, most of the time. The baby has a palmar grasp which is an automatic reaction and during the third month of life, brings the hands towards the midline (Case-Smith, 2006). Until three months of age, the baby's shoulder is adducted and close to the body, as the shoulder stability has not developed (Tecklin, 2008).

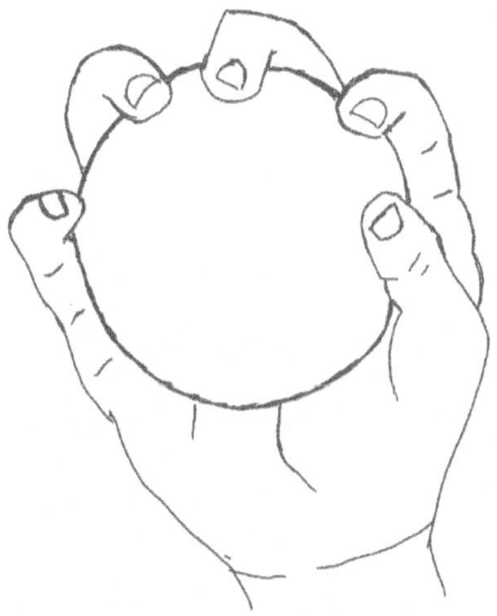

Palmar Grasp

Between three and five months, the baby can hold the trunk and lift the head off the surface. It leans on the forearms and hands to get support (Green, 2009). The baby begins to open the hands and is also able to put hands around the object. When lying on the back, the baby can touch the toys or objects that are presented to it. The baby is now able to move arms in a wider range and also develop an awareness of the hands in space (Bole, 2007).

Between six and seven months, the baby will have a stable trunk and is capable of moving the arms and legs independently. They can use their hands and arms to prop up and stabilize their trunk (Illingworth, 2007). The baby also learns to rotate forearm and wrist. The baby tries to crawl on hands and knees. Having visual regard and eye-hand coordination, the baby can explore the environment. The baby can move the thumb out of the palm but has a raking grasp. The baby can grasp an object when placed in his hands.

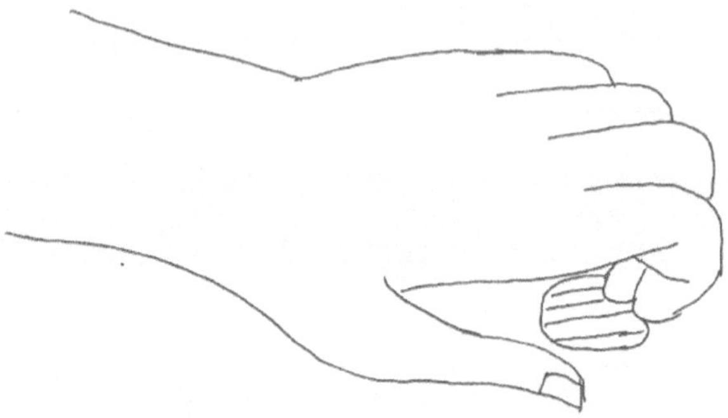

Raking grasp

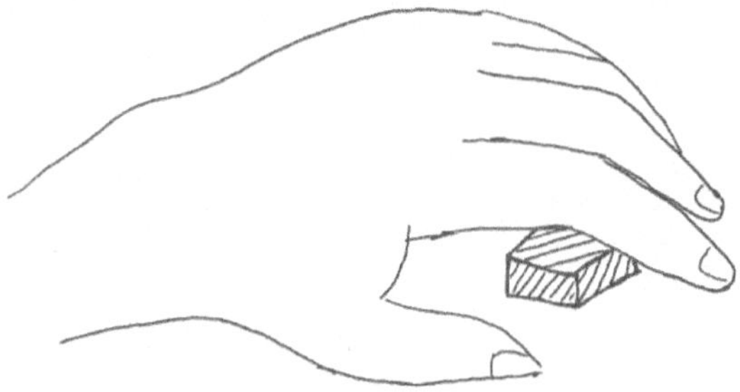

Raking grasp

Between seven and nine months of age, the baby can sit independently, shift weight in sitting and begin to rotate the trunk. The baby can support with one arm while sitting and use the other arm for reaching activities. They can hold objects with both hands and can rotate the forearm to drop objects from the hands. They can transfer objects from one hand to the other (Levitt, 2019) and also hold objects between thumb and forefingers fingers (radial grasp) while keeping the wrist in extension.

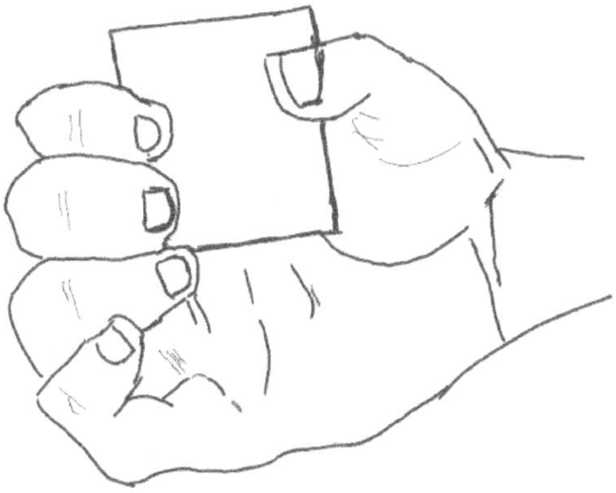

Radial grasp

Between nine and twelve months of age, the baby can stabilize the shoulder (Green, 2009) for reaching and grasping activities. They can reach and grasp in all directions (Levitt, 2019). They now have more precise control to grasp objects in hand, and to drop them. They can hold objects between thumb and index finger (pincer grasp) and also place the objects into containers. They achieve prewriting skills (Green, 2009).

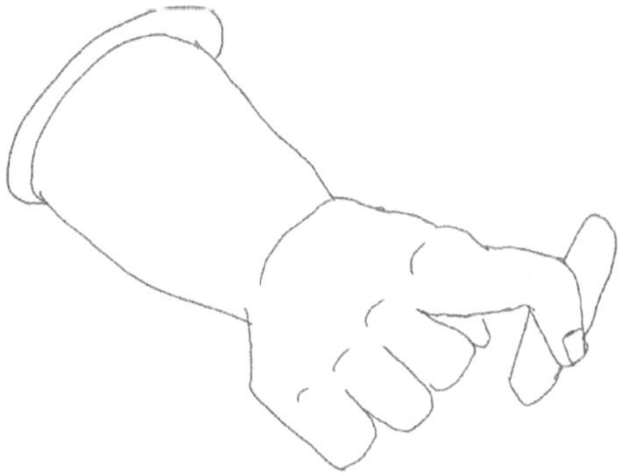

Pincer grasp

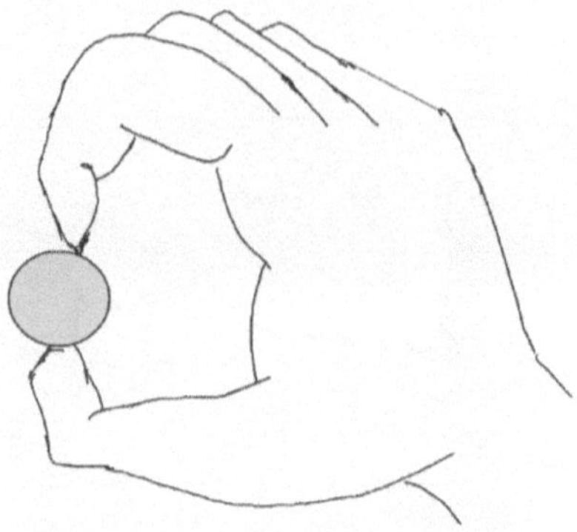

Pincer grasp

TYPICAL DEVELOPMENT OF HAND FUNCTIONS BETWEEN SECOND AND FIFTH YEAR OF LIFE

During the second year of life (12-24 months), the child can throw the ball but fall when doing so (Illingworth, 2007), scribble spontaneously, place pegs into holes and remove them. They can also turn pages, use a spoon, and open the little box. They hold objects between thumb and other fingers and also develop pincer grasp and release. They can build a tower of two to six cubes (Folio and Fewell, 2000).

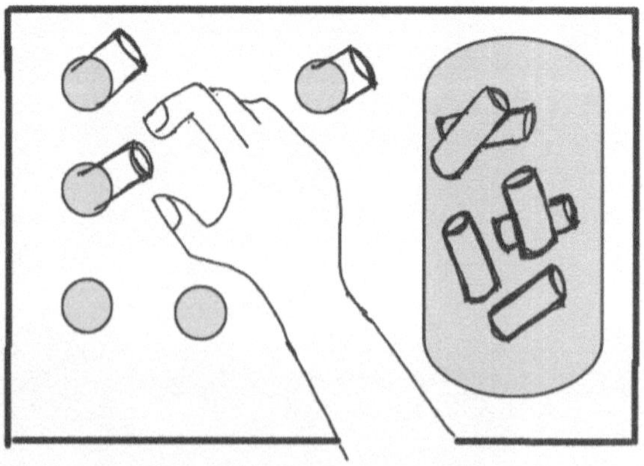

Child removing pegs from pegboard

During the third year of life (24-36 months), the child develops hand preference. They develop finger to palm translation and palm to finger translation. They can put pellets into bottles, copy horizontal line, vertical line, and circle (Illingworth, 2007). The child can catch a large ball with extended arms. They can also build a tower of six to eight cubes (Brown et al, 1981). The child can turn several pages of a book at a time (Folio and Fewell, 2000).

During the fourth year of life (36-48 months), the child can build a tower of nine blocks and identify different textures. In addition to copying a horizontal line, vertical line, circle, and a cross (X), the child can draw a man. The child may develop a static tripod grasp (Smith, 2001).

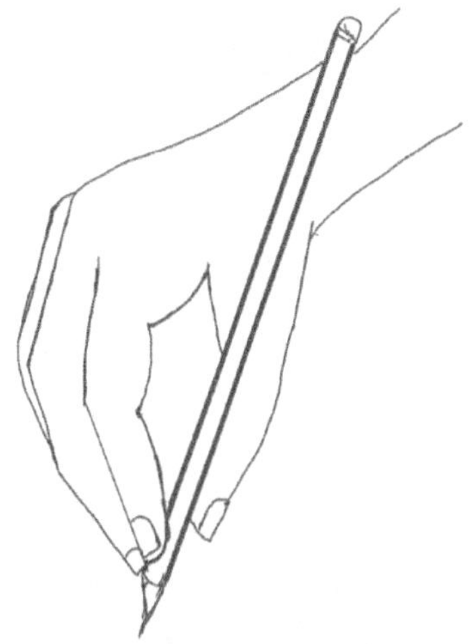

Static Tripod Grasp

They can identify objects such as a teaspoon, pencil, coins, and similar objects when placed in hand without looking at them. They can solve simple picture puzzles. The child can walk with the arms swinging in coordination with the opposite leg (Furuno et al, 2001).

During the fifth year of life (48-60 months), the child has good arm-leg coordination and can stabilize paper with one hand while using the other hand for writing. The child develops a tripod grip, and an open web space, while holding a pencil. The child can copy square, X, triangle and block letters (Levitt, 2019). When a coin is placed in palm the child can move the coin from the palm to fingers without placing them on the table (palm to finger translation).

CHAPTER 3: EVALUATION OF HAND FUNCTION

The evaluation of hand function in children with cerebral palsy involves a detailed assessment of the ability in performing daily activities such as the grasping of objects, releasing and the manipulation of the objects. Appropriate assessment of the hand function is crucial in the understanding of the status relating to the extent of the limitation in the hand function of the child and also will help in tailoring the exercises required for improving the child's ability in everyday activities (Sabapathy & Bhardwaj, 2011).

There are several tools or scales available that help to measure or quantify the function of the hand, evaluate the areas of deficit in hand performance and also to track the progress of the hand function and modify the exercises as applicable.

There are several methods to evaluate a child's hand function which include,

- Standardized assessments such as using scales ex. Motor assessment scale, Assisting Hand Assessment
- Clinical observation: Providing various activities to the child and observing the use of hand
- Developmental stages: Assessing the development of hand use across different age groups
- Functional classifications: Assessing the spontaneous use of hands in daily activities

The therapist should make a detailed assessment to understand the abilities of the child and to find the missing components that are required for optimal hand functioning. The dominance of the hand should be observed, and also the resting position of the upper limb. The position of the shoulder (protracted, retracted, or abducted), elbow (extended or flexed), wrist (flexed, extended, radial deviation or ulnar deviation), hand (clenched or open), thumb (cortical, abducted or adducted) and fingers (flexed interphalangeal joints) and range of motion of the joints should be noted.

The muscle tone of the child can be assessed by observing the attitude of the upper limbs, palpating the muscle with the thumb and forefinger, resistance to passive movements (Illingworth, 2007), and shaking of the limbs. The attitude of the upper limbs should be observed during movement while changing positions as well as when the limb is in position. The therapist can hold the upper limb above the wrist and shake it gently and rapidly. The baby with spasticity will have less movement, while the one with hypotonia will demonstrate more movement. The baby with severe spasticity has their hands clenched.

The Modified Ashworth scale can be used to measure the resistance to passive stretching of soft tissue. Measurement of spasticity according to the Modified Ashworth Scale (Bohannon and Smith, 1987) is as follows:

0 (No increase in muscle tone)

1 (Slight increase in muscle tone, manifested by a catch and release or by minimal resistance at the end of the range of motion when the affected part is moved in flexion or extension)

1+ (Slight increase in muscle tone, manifested by a catch, followed by minimal resistance throughout the remaining of the range of motion)

2 (More marked increase in muscle tone through most of the Range of Motion (ROM), but the affected parts easily moved)

3 (Considerable increase in muscle tone, making passive movement difficult)

4 (Affected parts are rigid in flexion or extension)

The child should be provided with different play toys, and activities to understand the manipulative skills, type of grasp and release, reaching patterns, the accuracy of reaching, coordination, and hand actions. The muscle length, muscle weakness, and presence of any contractures and deformities have to be assessed in more detail.

Communication level of the child plays an important role in the ability of the child to cooperate for therapy. It is important to see if the child has bilateral integration, presence of any abnormal reflexes, tremors, or involuntary movements.

The sensory system should be evaluated in terms of light touch, pain, temperature, deep pressure, stereognosis, and 2-point discrimination. The therapist should observe if the child enjoys or dislikes any particular sensations. For example, the child may cry on being dressed in clothes of certain materials. Neglect and disuse of the limb will be more if the sensory deficit is greater (Heest, House & Putnam 1993). Also, the motor impairment in the child is believed to be more if the sensory deficit is more (Kinnucan, Heest & Tomhave, 2010). Based on the above-mentioned factors, the therapist plans the treatment accordingly.

Some children having sensory processing disorders may exhibit emotional symptoms and these emotions may present as frustrations, impulsiveness, avoidance of eye contact, throwing tantrums. These children may struggle to express themselves, often feeling anxious and may withdraw from other children to play alone. These children will need a lot of reassurance from parents, therapists, and other caregivers (Sabapathy & Bhardwaj, 2011).

IDENTIFYING COMMON PATTERNS OF POOR HAND FUNCTION

It is quite important to know as to why a child is unable to perform a particular task, and identify components that prevent him from reaching the respective developmental milestones. Then, the therapist should work on the missing components to enable movement of the child. Some of the common patterns of poor hand function are mentioned below,

- Reaching for an object with wrist flexion

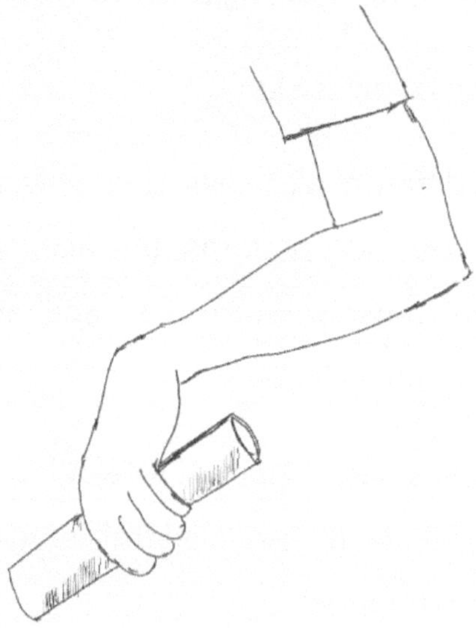

Wrist flexion with palmar grasp

- Excessive finger flexion when trying to grasp objects

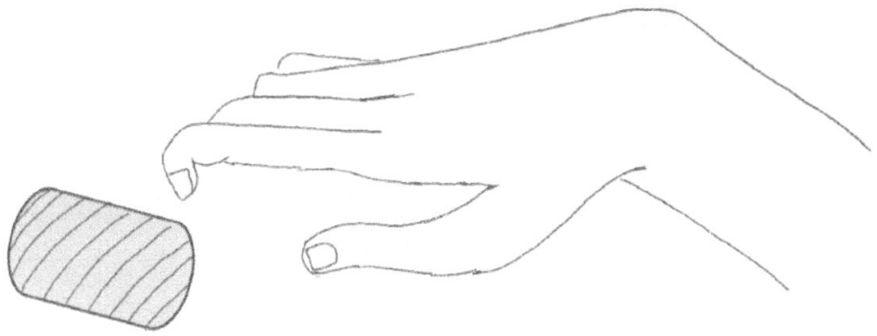

Excessive finger flexion during grasp

- Adducted thumbs
- Ulnar grasp

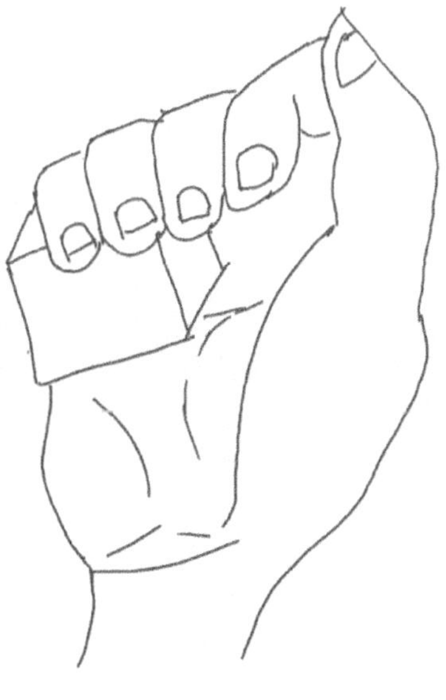

Ulnar Grasp

- Clenching hands when trying to grasp
- Bringing arms close to the body with elbows bent and the wrist in flexion (wrist bent such that the palm faces downwards) when trying to grasp
- When one hand tries to grasp an object, the other hand also clenches involuntarily

- Inability to let go of the object present in hand
- Able to let go of the object only with wrist flexion
- Release object with excessive splaying of fingers (hyperabduction with hyperextension at metacarpophalangeal joints)
- Thumb held in the palm
- Delay in grasping an object when placed in the hand
- Delay in reaching in all directions
- Inability to use both hands simultaneously
- Delay in transferring the object from one hand to the other
- Delay in finger-thumb opposition
- Unable to rotate the forearm so that the palm faces upwards (supination)
- The abduction of the arm with internal rotation makes the child over-pronate the forearm for hand use, which does cause a limitation in supination of the forearm.

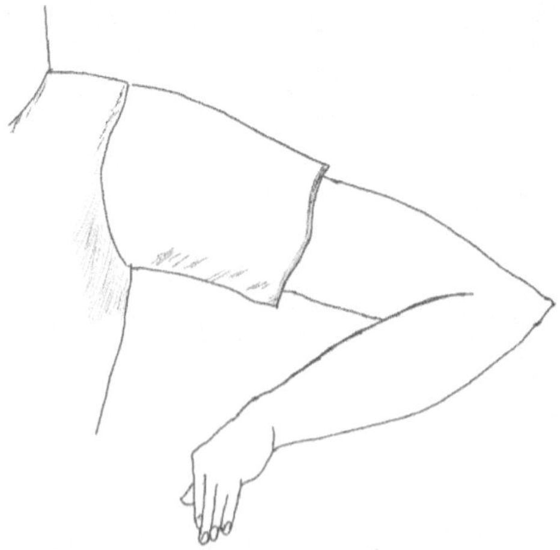

Arm abducted and internally rotated, elbow flexed and forearm pronated

A school-based checklist for a child involves identifying skills including gross grasp, palmar grasp, pincer grasp, and tripod grasp. The skills such as ability to isolate fingers, opening webspace, arch development in the hand, and thumb opposition play an important role in assessing the child's readiness for school inclusion. Also, the ability of separating the radial and ulnar function of the hand, and manipulation skills such as translation, shift and rotation are important. These skills will be elaborately explained in later chapters of this book. Other advanced skills for pencil grasp and handwriting that needs assessment include the ability to grasp, draw and write, dominance of hand, speed of writing and copying words, letters and shapes.

HAND FUNCTION EVALUATION SCALES

There are several hand function and evaluation scales used by therapists around the world. The commonly used scales are mentioned below:

Melbourne Assessment of Unilateral Upper Limb Function Test

Functional Independence Measure for Children (WeeFIM)

Peabody Developmental motor scales-2

Jebsen Hand Function Test

Abilhand-kids

Assisting Hand Assessment

Quality Upper Extremity Skill Test

The **Melbourne Assessment of the Unilateral Upper Limb Function Test** is widely used by the therapists as it demonstrates moderate to high consistency (Santos et al., 2015). The Quality Upper Extremity Skill test demonstrates good applicability of the test as well as performance. QUEST has 4 segments that evaluate dissociated movement, grasp, protective extension and weight-bearing (Ferreira et al., 2017). It is used in children from eighteen months to eight years of age (Hickey & Ziviani, 1998).

The **Peabody Developmental Motor Scale-2** is designed to evaluate gross and fine motor skills of children from birth to 72 months of age (Folio & Fewell, 2000). It has six subtests which include, reflexes, stationary (ability to sustain control of the body within its center of gravity and retain equilibrium), locomotion, object manipulation (child's movements required to throw and catch objects), grasping (ability to use hands starting from holding an object and subsequently progressing to controlled use of fingers), and visual-motor integration.

The **WeeFIM** can be used in children with disabilities and delays over seven years of age (Slomine, 2011). It has an 18-item performance measurement system that documents activities of self-care, functional mobility, as well as cognitive abilities. The self-care domain consists of eight items which include eating, grooming, bathing, lower and upper body dressing, toileting, as well as bowel and bladder control. The mobility domain consists of five items which include chair, toilet, and tub transfers, walking or wheelchair management, and stairs. The cognitive domain consists of five items which include language comprehension and expression, social interaction, problem-solving, and memory. It was used to measure the outcome and change in functional status over time.

Assisting Hand Assessment is used in children with unilateral disabilities, who have one hand functioning well while the other is less functioning (Krumlinde-Sundholm, Holmefur, Kottorp & Eliasson, 2007). It is commonly used in children with spastic hemiplegia or brachial plexus injury. Abilhand-kids is used to measure the manual ability in children with cerebral palsy. They are used to help in goal setting and planning of treatment. It is used widely in clinical practice (Arnould, Penta, Renders & Thonnard, 2004).

Jebsen-Taylor Hand Function Test is used to measure the level of hand function in children six years and above. It is simple, and a convenient method of administration. It has a seven-part timed diagnostic test. The test comprises of writing, turning cards, lifting small objects, simulated feeding, stacking, lifting large, lightweight and heavyweight objects (Culicchia et al., 2016). Usually, the non-dominant hand is tested first followed by the dominant hand. Each subtest is timed using a stopwatch. It is a simple tool to monitor the child's progress during therapy.

CHAPTER 4: PREPARING THE CHILD FOR HAND THERAPY AND FUNCTIONAL ACTIVITIES

The child with cerebral palsy may have several impairments including abnormalities of speech and language, perceptual defects, difficulties in recognizing objects or symbols (agnosia). The child may have language and visuomotor defects. This book is mainly focused on developing and improving the hand function of children with spastic cerebral palsy who have motor defects. The child with cerebral palsy sometimes in addition to motor defects may have associated perceptual defects and intellectual retardation. This is because of the lack of movements in these children, prevents them from exploring the environment. This lack of movements can affect the child's ability even in terms of language development. Thus, it is important to recognize the functions; the child is unable to perform and to treat the child accordingly. This book can be useful to teach the parents and caregivers of the child, some of the techniques that could be implemented in their homes to improve the functional ability of the child with cerebral palsy concerning their hand function.

The following principles are considered during the treatment of a child with cerebral palsy:

- The child needs motivation, the therapist/parent should take efforts in understanding the child's interest and use is it in the child's best interest to help the child focus on the task at hand
- Breaking tasks into several small steps will make the child learn the activity with ease
- Providing frequent rest periods between activities
- The child should be placed comfortably so that his concentration is not directed in adjusting himself to keep his trunk stable, thereby helping him to focus on his activity with hands.
- Length of the treatment should be planned according to the child's attention span
- Keeping distractions away from the room used for treatment
- Placing a hand over the child's body area, gentle vibrations can be provided. The application of the vibration should be consistent and comfortable to the child.

- Tapping over the muscle belly helps to initiate a voluntary contraction. According to Rood, tapping over the muscle belly 3 to 5 times facilitates movement.
- Slow stroking over the paravertebral muscles helps to inhibit muscle tone
- Slow and smooth passive movements within the comfortable and pain-free range will also help reduce muscle tone.
- Rapid oscillatory movements of the upper limb can inhibit the stiffness before activities.
- It is important to check if the child is well positioned and supported at his trunk and pelvis. The movement of the hands, arm, and shoulder activities such as reaching, involve postural adjustment (movement of the trunk) and hence it is important to keep the trunk and pelvis stable while training the child for hand function.
- The neck of the child should also be adequately supported to enhance eye-hand coordination. (if the child has poor head control)
- Repetition and consistent practice are essential to train the child in any new task

CHAPTER 5: THERAPEUTIC INTERVENTION TO IMPROVE HAND FUNCTION

Proximal control is motor control in that part of the body which is proximal to the body part that moves or performs an activity. Trunk is proximal to arm, elbow is proximal to hand, wrist is also proximal to hand etc... When the child is moving the arm, and then the proximal part of the body which is the trunk should have good control in terms of movement and posture. If the trunk has poor control, then the movement of the arm is affected as it does not provide a stable base for mobility in the distal body part. Similarly, when we talk about movement or function in the hands, then wrist becomes the proximal part and should have good control and provide stability so that hand function would be efficient. For proper function in the distal part of the body the proximal control and stability is essential. In children, when we prefer to work on reaching or hand function, and the child does not have adequate trunk control, and then the trunk should be well supported before initiating reaching/hand function.

According to Exner (2006), the areas that need to be considered during an intervention for hand skill development are, proper position of the child and the therapist, muscle tone and proximal control of the body part, tactile and sensory awareness, discrimination, isolated movement of arms and legs, grasping skills, in-hand manipulation, bilateral hand skill development, and integration of hand function skills into their respective occupations.

The important voluntary functions of the hand include the following:

Reach

Grasp

Release

Manipulation skills

Hand function, as well as the upper limb movement training, should be practiced in certain positions as described below. The position to be used depends on the age and the developmental level of the child.

IDEAL POSITIONS FOR DIFFERENT DEVELOPMENTAL LEVELS USED FOR TRAINING IN HAND FUNCTION

Between birth and three months, the infant is in supine lying. The infant can be encouraged to look at bright toys, ribbons, and rattles tied such that they are hanging above the child. This will encourage play behaviour. By three months of age, the grasp reflex (the baby will clench hands when the palm is touched) integrates and the baby will begin to open the hands. Between three to five months, the baby may be positioned in side-lying, supine, or prone, bearing weight on elbows with toys placed in front of the child to reach for. It would be ideal to train the baby to reach and grasp after the baby is 5 months old. Until five months of age, the baby should be presented with bright coloured toys to explore. The baby can be encouraged to hold rubber toys, large rings, and rattles.

Between six and eight months, the baby can be placed in sitting with hands propped in the front, and then, on the side (one hand propped). The baby can be propped on one hand (if the baby can stabilize its position) while reaching for toys with the other. The positions in side-lying and prone on elbows can also be used to encourage the baby to reach for toys. Rolling should be encouraged as it will develop upper limb patterns (shoulder flexion, adduction, and external rotation) that are required for reaching activities.

Between eight and ten months, the baby can be positioned on hands and knees (on fours) in addition to sitting. On fours, the baby will shift weight between hands and knees, enabling postural control. This position will also improve the stability of the shoulder girdle and at the pelvis. It will also improve the proprioceptive input at the joints. The baby will now be able to sit without support and use both hands to play with the toys. Between 7 to 10 months, the child can be encouraged to release an object, by placing the heel of the hand on the surface of the table or hard surface. After 7 months of age, the baby should be involved in transferring toys or objects from one hand to the other. Between ten and twelve months, the baby can be trained for reaching and grasping in upright kneeling and standing, if the child is comfortable and able to stabilize himself in these positions. Between 9 to 12 months of age, the child can pick up small objects such as beans, food, buttons, old crayons, pencils, chalk, etc...For children over 12 months, the reaching and grasping activities can be trained either in standing or sitting.

In any position, the child should be well supported to begin hand training. A corner chair can help the child to provide adequate support, as there would be enough space for the child to practice manipulative skills. The child's palm should be exposed to different sensations by rubbing different textures like sand, rice, soft cloth, sponges, velvet cloth, water, and so on. The baby/child should first be trained using light objects before introducing them to heavy objects. The child should be encouraged to actively rub hands on the face, arms and fee. The baby's wrists can be tied with colourful and bright bracelets or bells to motivate the baby to move the hands for activities such as reaching.

WEIGHT-BEARING ON EXTENDED ARMS

The baby/child depending on developmental level (ability to sit) can be made to sit with hands propped in front for a few minutes, then hands propped on either side and later with hands propped slightly behind the baby. The elbows must be maintained in extension while doing so. If the child cannot hold his elbows in extension, elbow gaiters/straps can be used to maintain elbows in extension. If the child's hands are clenched, apply mild pressure over the heels of the hands to open the child's hands, and then the thumb should be slowly moved out from its base. Mild pressure can be applied over the flat hands to keep them in position.

The child can be slightly tilted to either side, to enable weight shifting on hands. Alternately depending on the developmental level of the child, the child can be positioned on hands and knees or standing depending on his /her developmental level. The therapist or caregiver of the child can provide adequate support for the child to maintain the position. This applies a prolonged stretch on the forearm muscles with the child, weight-bearing on the hands, thus providing adequate stretch on the forearms, helping in better upper limb flexibility.

When the child is on hands and knees, the therapist should take care that the hips and shoulders are at right angles. The hands should slightly turn outwards to avoid internal rotation. If the child needs support, he can also be positioned in prone on a bolster (on fours), such that the bolster supports the trunk. This position helps in improving trunk control and shoulder stability. The child can be provided with toys so that the child support with one hand, while playing with the other. Also, the child gets appropriate proprioceptive input through weight-bearing.

Reaching should be practiced by providing toys to the child, starting first from low down in front of the child, then forward at shoulder level. When the child is comfortable, then, reaching should be encouraged from the side of the child, followed by, above the shoulder level and later from slightly behind the child (Levitt 2019).

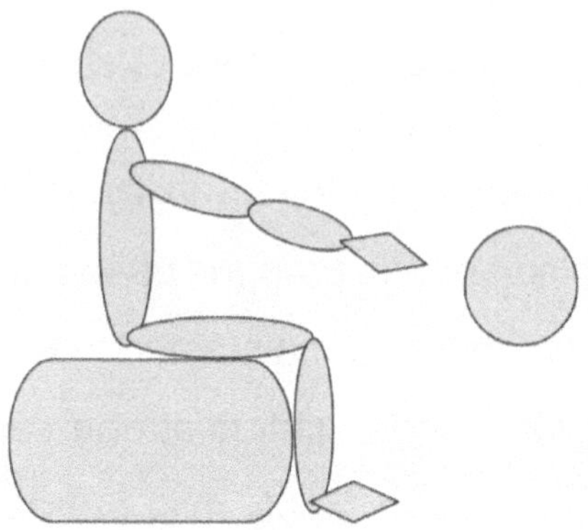

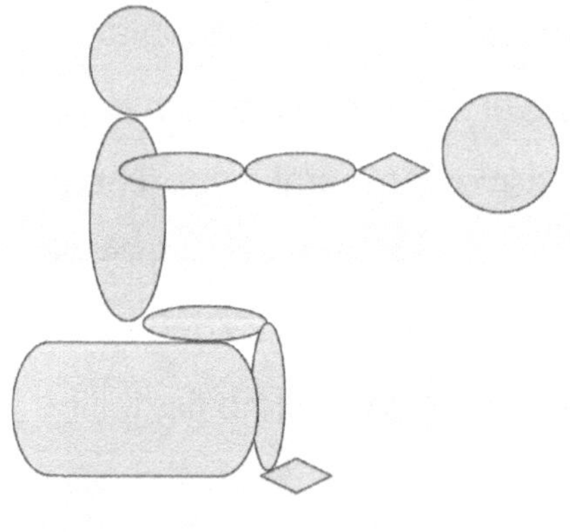

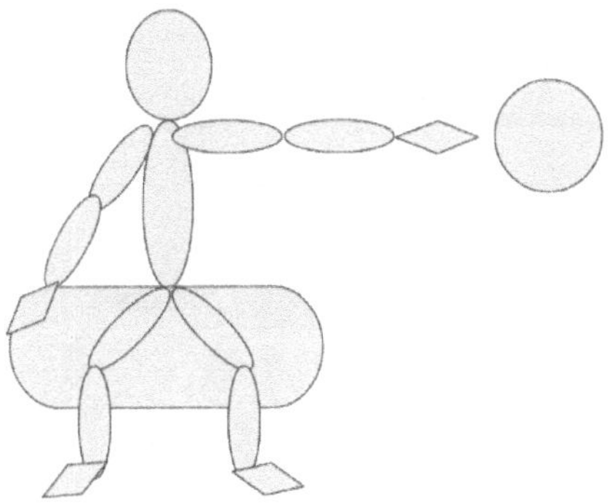

This could most probably be due to the fact that the child develops weight shifting first in the anterior-posterior direction, then lateral weight shifts, and finally the ability to rotate. In some children, we may need to train reaching first in sideways (laterally) to enable shoulder adduction, which is an important component in reaching activities. In such cases, we can train reaching within the base of support, so the child does not require shifting weight to reach.

If the child has his hands always clenched, there could be problems with the opening of his hands when letting go of objects from his hands. A soft cone or anti-spasticity cone can be placed in the child's hands if there is difficulty in opening the hands for grasp. The anti-spasticity cone is made of firm material and covered with thermoplastic material. The large end of the anti-spasticity cone should be towards the side of the little finger while the small end towards the thumb. This allows more contact of the cone with the palm and inhibits spasticity by applying deep pressure on the flexor tendons and muscles. This improves opening the hands for children who have fisting or clenched hands. Do not give the child toys or objects that get squeezed on holding. Soft cones may be given in children who have fisting that the fingers dig into the palm. Once some amount of hand opening is established, then the anti-spasticity cone can be used.

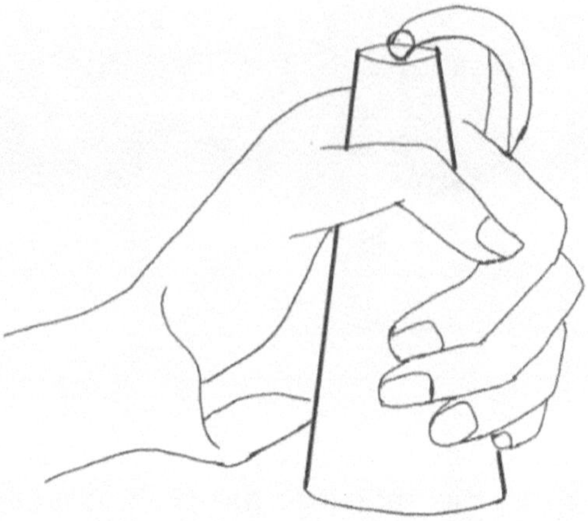

Anti-spasticity cone

If the child grasps or holds an object/toy with the wrist in flexion, the therapist or the caregiver should press the child's wrist or dorsum forearm down, as he tries to grasp the toy. Then the therapist should try placing the object either in line with the wrist or slightly higher than the level of his wrist so that the child is asked to lift his hand to the object. A wrist splint can also be used to accomplish this technique. The child should be encouraged to do activities such as removing pegs in a pegboard or removing rings off the cone.

Sometimes when the child uses one hand to hold or grasp an object, the other hand also clenches. To prevent this act, it would be recommended that the hand that is not in use should be placed flat on the table with some mild pressure over the hand when the child uses the other hand for activities. Alternately, the child is encouraged to put more weight on the hand that is placed flat on the table.

For children with spasticity or abnormal tone, supination is the most difficult movement to achieve. According to Exner (2006), most of the functional skills of the upper limb require the range of supination from full pronation to mid-position, where most skills using the radial fingers require the range of supination from 30 degrees to 45 degrees of supination. The intervention for improving the range of supination should be focused best by maintaining the arm in adduction and the elbow is flexed.

If the child tries to grasp the object with excessive finger flexion, then the therapist or the caregiver should place the child's hands over thick larger objects such as bars and handles. Care should be taken to not force the fingers into extension (Levitt, 2019). For children with difficulty in the voluntary opening of the hands, weight-bearing by placing the hands flat on the table can be encouraged. But this should be handled with care and caution as the child with this issue may not have the optimal length of the musculature in finger flexors. In these children, weight-bearing if possible can be tried on curved surfaces rather than flat surfaces. Also, the child should not be encouraged to bear full weight on their hands for fear of injury. The child can be encouraged to hold the edge of the card and turn the card.

If the child has his thumb adducted (thumb held close to palm), the forearm can be supinated, and then the thumb may be slowly taken out of the fist. Caution should be exercised when the thumb is slowly abducted from its base. Care should be taken not to force the thumb into abduction, as doing so may cause dislocation of the joint.

Children who hold toys with ulnar grasp will benefit if they are trained to grasp the objects/toys by moving the hands towards the thumb side. The therapist can hold the child's hand during grasp, such that the therapist places his thumb between the child's thumb and forefinger, and the rest of the therapist's fingers holds the ulnar side of the child's hands down (as shown in the picture below), thus encouraging radial grasp. The little finger and the ring finger of the child may be bandaged if the child finds it comfortable. Splints can be used to hold the thumb in abduction (away from palm) when not using hands.

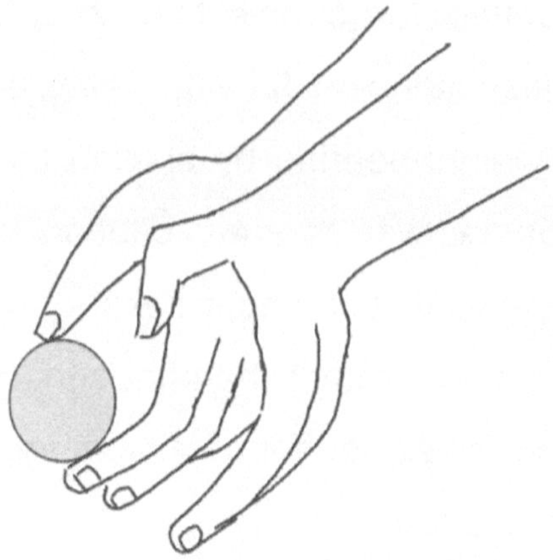

Therapist Guiding Thumb Abduction and Pincer Grasp

SWEEP TAPPING TO ENCOURAGE WRIST EXTENSION

Supporting the child's arm with one hand, using the other hand, sweep firmly and briskly from above the elbow over the origin of the extensor muscle group to fingertips. The sweeping movement is performed with the therapist's fingers held firmly in extension (Davies, 1985). After a few sweeps finger extension is possible. After sweep tapping, it is recommended to provide the child with activities to improve hand function.

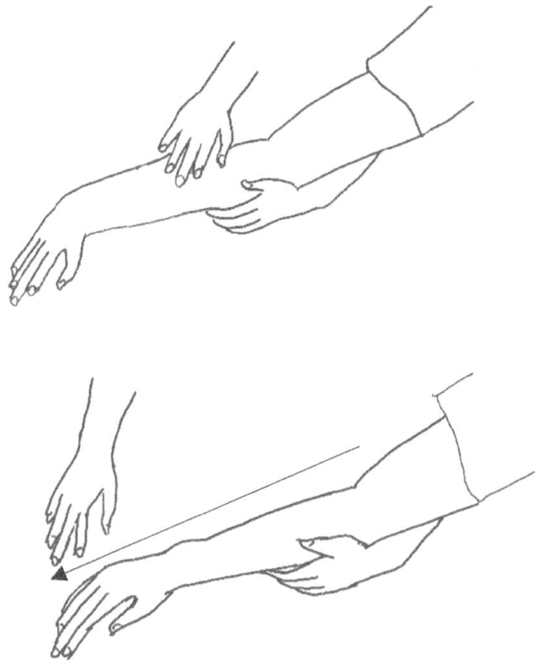

Sweep Tapping

THE VOLUNTARY RELEASE OF OBJECTS

Children who have difficulty releasing objects may have poor stability at the shoulder, or/and at the wrist. They may also have increased tone in the flexor musculature that causes their hands to clench or fist. It is a common pattern for children with cerebral palsy to grasp only with wrist flexion associated with elbow flexion. They may also voluntarily release the object with some wrist extension helped by simultaneous elbow flexion. Children having poor stability at the shoulder should be trained for voluntary release by keeping the arm close to the body. Also, they would benefit if they are trained in reaching activities to help develop shoulder stability. Children with poor wrist stability can release the objects effectively if their wrist is supported.

A common pattern in children with cerebral palsy is releasing an object with wrist flexion. The therapist or the caregiver should train to release the objects keeping the child's wrist in neutral or midline (in line with the forearm). A splint, manual support and active control of child if possible will provide additional support. Also, firm stroking on the back of the hand from the base of the fingers across the wrist will help in opening the fingers while releasing the objects into a container.

If the child releases the object in hand with thumb adducted and flexed in palm (Levitt, 2019): Training should be provided with child's active hand opening combined together with thumb abduction (movement of thumb away from the palm) following supination (rotation of forearm such that the palm is facing the ceiling) of forearm by therapist or caregiver.

We can stroke over the skin on the dorsum of the hand (the muscles for finger extension are present) starting from the base of the fingers across the wrist joint and continue to the lower end of the forearm. It is a stimulation technique that activates the sensory cortex and also helps to activate the muscles over the dorsum of the hand which is responsible for opening of the fingers (the extension of the fingers).

If the child releases the object in hand with thumb adducted and flexed in palm (Levitt, 2019), training should be provided with child's active hand opening combined together with thumb abduction (movement of thumb away from the palm) following supination (rotation of forearm such that the palm is facing the ceiling) of forearm by therapist or caregiver.

If the child releases the object in hand with ulnar deviation (hand deviated towards the side of the little finger), hand training should be provided such that the objects are released into a container or dowel holes on radial side (thumb side) of hands.

Shaking the child's arm rhythmically from the shoulder will play a great role to relax the child's hand. This technique has proven to be invaluable in my practice with children with cerebral palsy. Also stroking the ulnar surface of the child's hand and little finger will help in opening the hand. The child can be allowed to weight bear when lying prone on elbows, or sit by weight-bearing on hands (hands flat) with extended elbows on a table, to help in an active hand opening.

If the above techniques do not help then, the child's arms can be rotated outwards or the forearm supinated to ease the hand opening especially when releasing the objects. The child should be placed in a comfortable position, when training for hand function, and reaching should be encouraged past his midline for reaching objects.

Encourage the child to throw and catch a big ball with both hands, this develops bilateral integration. The child can be provided with a softball that can be squeezed. The strength of the intrinsic muscles in hand improves. The child should be encouraged to hold objects of different sizes and weights into the hands.

In-hand manipulation meaning 'manipulation of the objects within the hand' comprises of moving or adjusting the objects within the hand. They include finger to palm translation (object is moved from the fingers to the palm), palm to finger translation (object is moved from the palm to the fingers), shift (adjustment of the object within the hand using the finger pads), simple rotation (slight rotation of the objects with the fingers less than 90 degrees) and complex rotation (rotation of the object in the hand with fingers more than 90 degrees and less than 360 degrees) (Exner, 1992). Initially, the child before developing the skills of in-hand manipulation tries to stabilize or adjust the object within the hand using supporting surface. The child is encouraged to play with objects that are not too big or too small for the child's hands.

CRITERIA TO IMPROVE IN-HAND MANIPULATION SKILLS:

Children should be well trained in the reach, grasp, and release of objects and capable of supination of the forearm at least to mid-position for them to be able to manipulate the objects within the hand. They should have adequate control of the intrinsic musculature of the hand, and independent finger movements to be able to hold the objects for manipulation.

ACTIVITIES TO IMPROVE IN-HAND MANIPULATION SKILLS

The child may be encouraged to play with small coins or pegs, asking them to pick them with the fingers and transfer to the palm. Once the child can handle this skill efficiently, palm to finger translation can be encouraged, where the therapist places the object in the palm asking the child to move it to the fingers and drop them in a container. Simple rotation can be encouraged by asking the child to place pegs in a pegboard, where the child rotates the peg to bring it to the position before placing it on the pegboard or picking a pencil and holding between the thumb and forefingers. Children with mild disability are capable of being trained for in-hand manipulation skills.

When using a pegboard to place and remove pegs, the child can be encouraged to first use the thumb and the index finger, then thumb and middle finger, thumb and ring finger, and later thumb and little finger to handle the pegs. This will improve the use of independent finger movements, using the thumb in coordination with the other fingers.

The child can be given a picture puzzle and asked to solve it. Clay moulding can be encouraged, as moulding the clay into different geometrical figures helps to strengthen the intrinsic muscles of the hand. The child can pick pasta or cereals with the fingers and hold it in the palm or put them into a container. Finger painting would be a fun activity for the child, motivating them for skilled use of their fingers. The child can also be provided with finger foods to encourage picking small items with the fingers.

OTHER FINE MOTOR SKILLS AND ACTIVITIES

Activities to open thumb space: Encouraging the child to squeeze a soft ball or a clothespin with the thumb and the index finger will help to keep the thumb web space open.

Arch development: Children can be encouraged to crumble papers making it into a ball and throwing it onto a specified target.

Distal joint dexterity: Putting beads into string, colouring with crayons, playing with paperclips, tearing paper into bits, stacking coins and similar activities canhelp improve distal dexterity

Separation of the sides of the hand: One of the crucial skills in the development of hand includes the promotion of separation of both sides of the hand during different tasks. One side of the hand is used for stabilizing while the other is used for precision activities as writing, buttoning and so on…

The aim of using orthosis is to maintain the anatomical and functional position of the body part. They can be quite helpful in preventing contractures and deformities. There are static and dynamic orthoses, depending on the functional assessment and needs of each child, which is highly variable. It would be required for the child to wear orthotics (if needed) for about 4 to 8 hours a day. Orthotics can help in stretching the muscles.

Always choose splints that are made of low-temperature materials and can be remodeled. The straps in the splints should not be too thin or tight as they can hurt the skin. Care should be taken to check the skin regularly for any irritation.

Elbow gaiters: To keep the elbows extended. This helps to prevent flexion contracture at the elbows, which is a common feature in cerebral palsy. Elbow gaiters can also be used when the child is unable to keep elbows extended with the hands flat on the table (propped up) during therapy. Proper padding should be provided in the forearm and care taken not to force the elbows or forearm into the splint.

Resting hand splint: To keep the wrist in an optimal position and prevent wrist flexion deformities. The resting hand splint is usually used in children with low tone, and minimal muscle tightness. In using the resting hand splints, the wrist and the fingers are extended to the maximum, within the comfort level of the child.

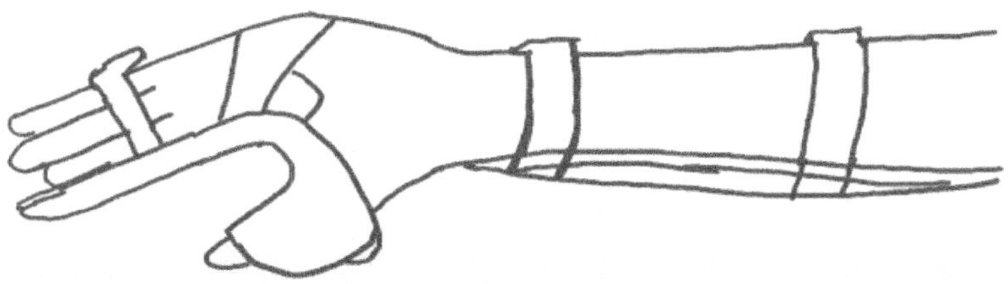

Resting hand splint

Prone wedges: To support the child in prone lying, and freeing the hands for hand training. They are usually made of moulded foam. They are soft and have straps to keep the child in position. They help to improve the child's tolerance to prone lying.

Dorsal splint: The dorsal splint covers more the dorsal part of the hands and forearm, and thus can be used for functional activities.

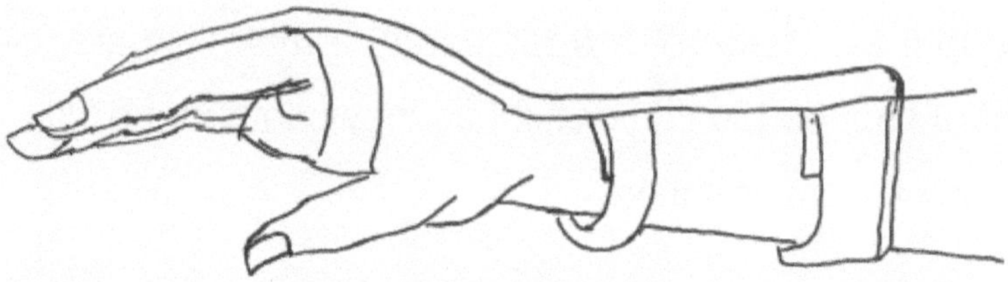

Dorsal splint

For children with less severe contractures, an inflatable hand splint can be provided. Some children may also need finger separators to keep the fingers in an optimal position.

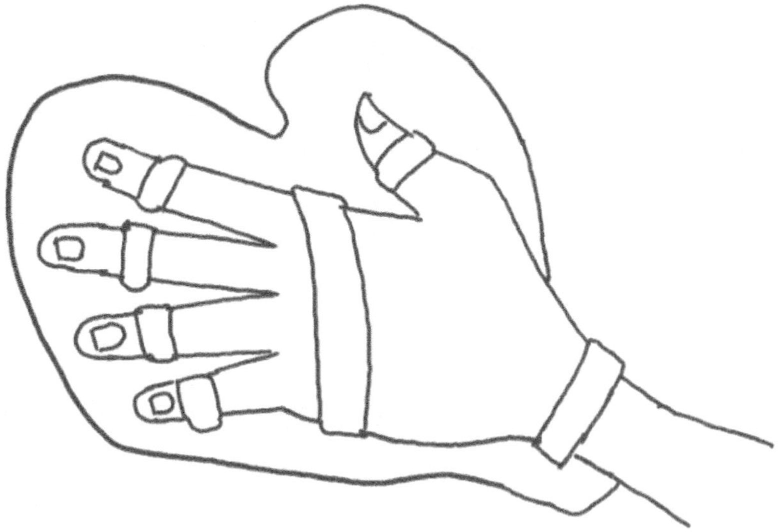

Finger Separator

Thumb abduction splint: Can be used in children who have a thumb in the palm. This orthotic can help the child to grasp or hold a toy, which cannot be achieved with the thumb in the palm. Care should be taken to avoid covering the skin much, to enable sensory feedback.

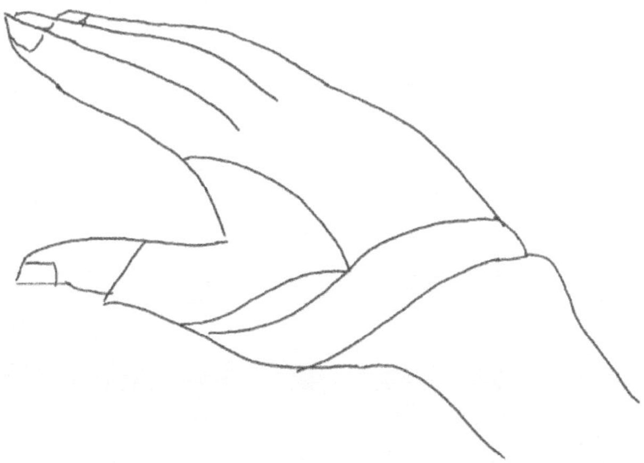

Thumb Abduction Splint

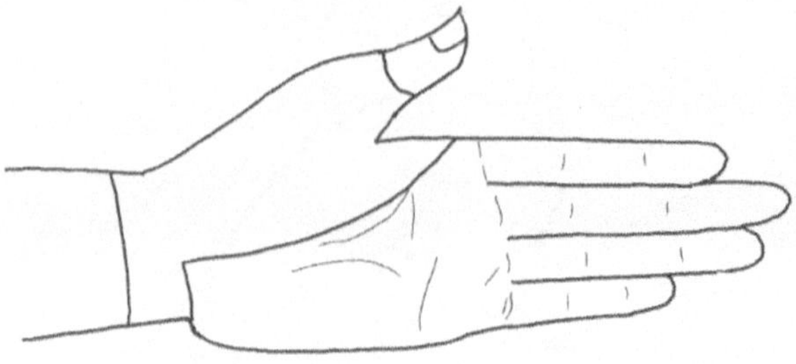

Thumb Abduction Splint

Swan neck splints: These splints are used when the proximal interphalangeal joint is hyperextended and the distal interphalangeal joint is flexed.

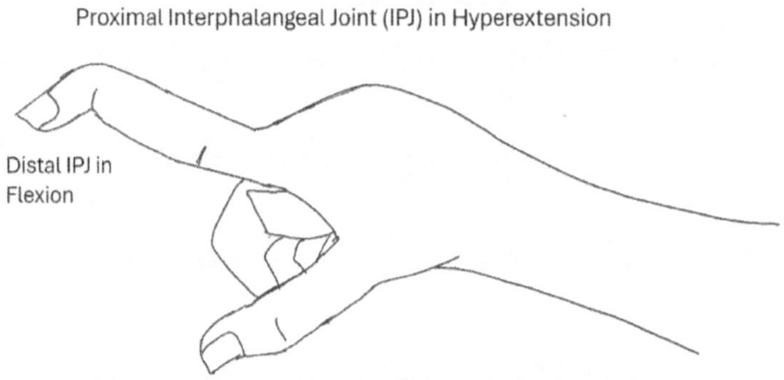

Swan Neck Deformity in Index Finger

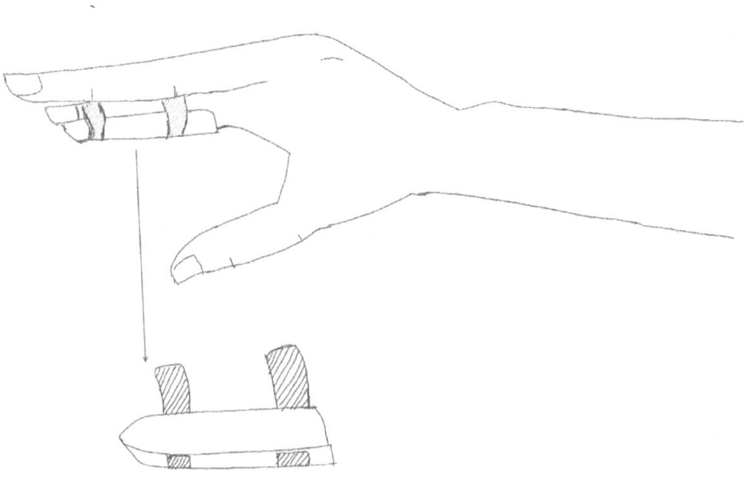

Splint for Swan Neck Deformity

Cerebral palsy chair: For children who are not yet able to sit without support, a specially designed chair can be used. The chair can be customized according to the child's needs. The chair has straps to keep chest and pelvis in place, providing adequate support. Some chairs also have head support with a strap for the forehead. The seat height of the chair will enable to keep the child's knee bent at 90 degrees. Lumbar support is provided to keep the normal lumbar lordosis. The feet should rest flat on the ground or a footrest. Supports can be placed on either side of the child's trunk to keep the trunk in position. Knee blocks help to keep the pelvis in position. A table can be attached to the chair, allowing the child for manipulative skills. The child should be trained to sit well back so that he takes weight equally on his hips, thighs, and feet.

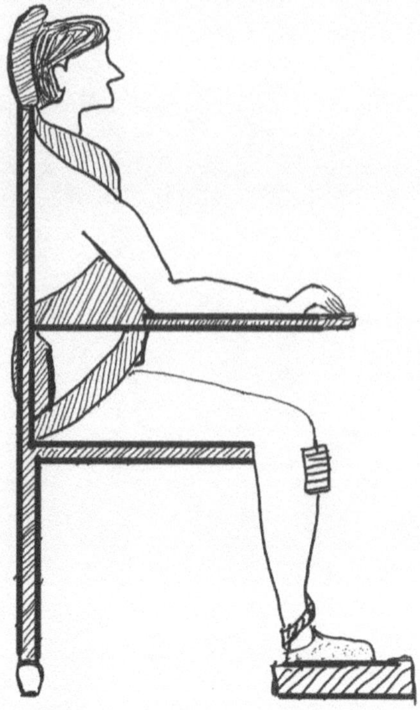

Special Chair With Supports

GLOSSARY

Abduction: The movement of a limb or other part away from the midline of the body, or from another part ("English Dictionary, Thesaurus, & Grammar Help | Lexico.com", 2019).

Adduction: The movement of a limb or other part towards the midline of the body or another part ("English Dictionary, Thesaurus, & Grammar Help | Lexico.com", 2019).

Contractures: Contracture is a fixed shortening of a muscle often leading to decreased joint range of movement.

Dynamic tripod grasp: In this grasp, the pencil rests on the middle finger, and the pads of the index and middle finger hold the pencil, to form a circle with the web space. Dynamic is the movement of the writing using the thumb, middle and index finger, with some movement at the wrist.

Extension: An unbending movement around a joint in a limb (such as the knee or elbow) that increases the angle between the bones of the limb at the joint ("Medical Dictionary by Merriam-Webster", 2019)

Flexion: A bending movement around a joint in a limb (such as the knee or elbow) that decreases the angle between the bones of the limb at the joint ("Medical Dictionary by Merriam-Webster", 2019)

Grasping reflex: When an object is placed in the palm, the infant holds the object tightly for a few seconds

Hand regard: The baby watches the movement of the hands when lying supine

Hypoxia: Deficiency of oxygen reaching the brain

Ischemia: Decreased supply of blood to a body part such as the brain (causing damage to the motor cortex)

Palmar grasp: The baby holds the objects in the palm and fingers for a few seconds to a minute

Paravertebral muscles: Muscles that are adjacent to the spinal column

Pincer grasp: Grasp of an object using the tips of the index finger and the thumb

Proprioceptive: Relating to stimuli that are produced and perceived within an organism, especially those connected with the position and movement of the body ("English Dictionary, Thesaurus, & Grammar Help | Lexico.com", 2019).

Perceptual: Of, relating to, or involving perception especially concerning immediate sensory experience ("Medical Dictionary by Merriam-Webster", 2019

Pronation: Rotation of the hand and forearm in a way that the palm faces downwards

Protraction: Movement of the scapula (shoulder blade) anterior and away from the spine. The shoulder thus moves forward

Raking grasp: The baby grasps by bending the fingers to bring the object closer into the hand

Reflex: An automatic and often inborn response to a stimulus that typically involves a nerve impulse passing inward from a receptor to the spinal cord and then passing outward from the spinal cord to an effector (such as a muscle or gland) without reaching the level of consciousness and often without passing to the brain. ("Medical Dictionary by Merriam-Webster", 2019)

Radial grasp: Pick or grasp an object using the middle finger, index finger, and the thumb

Retraction: Movement of the scapula (shoulder blade) posterior and towards the spine. The shoulder thus moves backwards

Spasticity: Hypertonicity of the muscle (increased muscle tone)

Spastic diplegia: A type of cerebral palsy, in which the lower limbs are more affected than the upper limbs.

Spastic hemiplegia: A type of cerebral palsy in which one side of the upper limb and the lower limb are affected.

Spastic quadriplegia: A type of cerebral palsy in which the upper limbs (bilateral) lower limbs (bilateral), including the neck and the trunk are affected.

Stereognosis: It is the ability to identify or perceive an object or a material by touching, holding or handling the object (tactile recognition).

Supination: Rotation of the forearm and hand such that the palm faces upwards

Ulnar grasp: Holding the objects with the ulnar or medial side of the palm

Vestibular system: System in the inner ear, responsible for the perception of body position and movement

Visual-perceptual: Ability of the brain to interpret what the child sees with the eyes.

REFERENCES

Abduction | Definition of abduction by Lexico. (2019). Retrieved 30 August 2019, from https://www.lexico.com/en/definition/abduction

Adduction | Definition of adduction by Lexico. (2019). Retrieved 30 August 2019, from https://www.lexico.com/en/definition/adduction

Arnould, C., Penta, M., Renders, A., & Thonnard, J. (2004). ABILHAND-Kids. Neurology, 63(6), 1045-1052. doi: 10.1212/01.wnl.0000138423.77640.37

Bohannon, R., & Smith, M. (1987). Interrater Reliability of a Modified Ashworth Scale of Muscle Spasticity. Physical Therapy, 67(2), 206-207. doi: 10.1093/ptj/67.2.206

Brown, S. L., D'Eugenio, D. B., Drews, J. E., Haskin, B. S., Lynch, E. W. Moersch, M. S., & Rogers, S. J. (1981). Preschool Developmental Profile (Vol. 5). Ann Arbor, MI: Michigan Press.

Case-Smith, J. (Ed.). (2001). Occupational therapy for children (4th ed.). St. Louis: Mosby.

Chu, S., Howard, L., Hume, C., & Hong, C. (2003). Occupational therapy in childhood (1st ed., pp. 129-147). London: Whurr.

Culicchia, G., Nobilia, M., Asturi, M., Santilli, V., Paoloni, M., De Santis, R., & Galeoto, G. (2016). Cross-Cultural Adaptation and Validation of the Jebsen-Taylor Hand Function Test in an Italian Population. Rehabilitation Research And Practice, 2016, 1-12. doi: 10.1155/2016/8970917

Davies, P. (1985). Steps to follow. Berlin: Springer-Verlag.

Definition of Extension. (2019). Retrieved 30 August 2019, from https://www.merriam-webster.com/dictionary/extension

Definition of Flexion. (2019). Retrieved 30 August 2019, from https://www.merriam-webster.com/dictionary/flexion

Definition of Perceptual. (2019). Retrieved 30 August 2019, from https://www.merriam-webster.com/dictionary/perceptual

Definition of Reflex. (2019). Retrieved 30 August 2019, from https://www.merriam-webster.com/dictionary/reflex

Dido Green. Hand function and fine motor activities. Chapter 19, Finnie's Handling the Young Child with Cerebral Palsy at Home (2009) Edition IV, Elsevier Ltd; pg 244-248.

Exner (1992). In hand manipulation skills. In J Case-Smith, C Pehoski, editors. Development of hand skills in the child (pp. 35-45). Rockville, MD. The American Occupational Therapy Association.

Exner, C. (2006). Hand function in the child: Foundations for remediation by Anne Henderson, Charlane Pehoski (2nd ed.). St. Louis, Mo.: Mosby/Elsevier.

Fell, D., Lunnen, K. and Rauk, R., 2018. Lifespan Neurorehabilitation. Philadelphia: F.A.Davis Company, p.493.

Ferreira, H., Cirne, G., Pereira, S., Lima, N., Cacho, R., & Cacho, E. (2017). Upper extremity motor quality evaluation in children with Cerebral Palsy. Fisioterapia Em Movimento, 30 (suppl 1), 277-284. doi: 10.1590/1980-5918.030.s01.ao27

Folio MR, Fewell RR (2000). Peabody developmental motor scale, second edition. Therapy skill builders, TX, 2000.

Furuno, S., O'Reilly, K., Inatsuka, T., Hosaka, C., Allman, T., & Zeisloft-Falbey, B. (1991). Hawaii Early Learning Profile. Palo Alto, CA: VORT.

Hickey, A., & Ziviani, J. (1998). A Review of the Quality of Upper Extremities Skills Test (QUEST) for Children with Cerebral Palsy. Physical & Occupational Therapy In Pediatrics, 18(3), 123-135. doi: 10.1300/j006v18n03_09

Kinnucan, Van Heest, Tomhave, Correlation of motor function and stereognosis impairment in the upper limb in cerebral palsy. Journal Hand Surg Am 2010; 35(8): 1317-1322

Krumlinde-Sundholm, L., Holmefur, M., Kottorp, A., & Eliasson, A. (2007). The Assisting Hand Assessment: current evidence of validity, reliability, and responsiveness to change. Developmental Medicine & Child Neurology, 49(4), 259-264. doi: 10.1111/j.1469-8749.2007.00259.x

L Andrew Koman, Beth Paterson Smith, J S Shilt, Cerebral Palsy, The Lancet, 2004, May 15, Vol 36

Levitt, S. (2019). Treatment of cerebral palsy and motor delay (6th ed.). Malden, MA: Blackwell.

Luzia Iara Pfeifer, Thaís Reis Santos, Daniela Baleroni Rodrigues Silva, Maria Paula Panúncio Pinto, Carla Andrea Caldas & Jair Lício Ferreira Santos (2014) Hand function in the play behaviour of children with cerebral palsy, Scandinavian Journal of Occupational Therapy, 21:4, 241-250, DOI: 10.3109/11038128.2013.871059

MacLennan, A., Thompson, S., & Gecz, J. (2015). Cerebral palsy: causes, pathways, and the role of genetic variants. American Journal Of Obstetrics And Gynecology, 213(6), 779-788. doi: 10.1016/j.ajog.2015.05.034

Miller, F., & Bachrach, S. J. (2006). Cerebral palsy: a complete guide for caregiving. 2nd ed. Baltimore: Johns Hopkins University Press.

O'Shea T. M. (2008). Diagnosis, treatment, and prevention of cerebral palsy. Clinical obstetrics and gynaecology, 51(4), 816–828. doi:10.1097/GRF.0b013e3181870ba7

Pitroda Nidhi, The effect of play therapy over conventional therapy in improving the hand function of spastic diplegic cerebral palsy children, Indian journal of physiotherapy and occupational therapy, 2008

Proprioceptive | Definition of proprioceptive by Lexico. (2019). Retrieved 30 August 2019, from https://www.lexico.com/en/definition/proprioceptive

Ronald, S.Illingworth (2007). Illingworth's The Development of the Infant and Young Child Normal and Abnormal. 9thed. Greater Noida, India: Elsevier

Bole Vijayalakshmi, Bole Suryakant. (2007). Early Management of Cerebral Palsy Including Children with Developmental Delays - A Practical Approach to Pediatric Occupational Therapy. 1st ed. Jaypee Brothers Medical Publisher (P) Ltd: Jitendar P Vij, pp.7-12.

Santos, C., Franco de Moura, R., Lazzari, R., Dumont, A., Braun, L., & Oliveira, C. (2015). Upper limb function evaluation scales for individuals with cerebral palsy: a systematic review. Journal Of Physical Therapy Science, 27(5), 1617-1620. doi: 10.1589/jpts.27.1617

Slomine, B. (2011). Functional Independence Measure for Children. Encyclopedia Of Clinical Neuropsychology, 1113-1115. doi: 10.1007/978-0-387-79948-3_1607

Case-Smith, Jane (2006), Hand skill development in the context of infant's play: Birth to 2 years, Hand function in the child: Foundations for remediation. Second edition. 117-137

Tecklin, J. (2008). Pediatric physical therapy (4th ed.). Philadelphia: Lippincott Williams & Wilkins.

Terence Y.P Chin, Josie A, Duncan et al, 2005, Management of Upperlimb in Cerebral Palsy, Journal of Paediatric Orthopaedics B. November 2005 - Volume 14 - Issue 6 - pp 389-404

Van Heest, House, Putnam. Sensibility deficiencies in the hands of children with spastic hemiplegia. J Hand Surgery Am. 1993; 18(2): 278-281

Sabapathy, Sr. and Bhardwaj, P. (2011) 'Assessment of the hand in cerebral palsy', *Indian Journal of Plastic Surgery*, 44(2), p. 348. doi:10.4103/0970-0358.85356.

Made in United States
Cleveland, OH
04 November 2026

47647263R00030